Foreword

The Royal College of Midwives and the Royal College of Obstetricians and Gynaecologists have welcomed the opportunity to work together on this guidance document which we believe clearly sets out our informed and considered views about the essential minimum midwife and medical staff numbers required to support women in labour.

This report acknowledges the increased involvement of the consultant obstetrician in the labour ward in the care of women with complex or complicated pregnancies and in the supervision and education of medical staff. The report pertains to the role of the midwife in secondary care settings and her central role as the expert autonomous practitioner in the care of women in normal labour. Together, obstetricians and midwives collaborate with anaesthetists and paediatricians in the care of women with complex and complicated labours.

In producing this document we were able to recognise and demonstrate the value of multidisciplinary and user involvement in delivering a comprehensive guide to improve interdisciplinary communication in order to improve organisation, practice and ultimately lead "Towards Safer Childbirth".

The recommendations and suggested auditable standards contained within the report will, we hope, inform Trusts and Health Authorities of the means to achieve improved standards of care for women in labour. In addition they will provide for medical staff and midwives the essential tools to support the continuing development of Clinical Governance.

Professor Robert Shaw
President RCOG

Mrs Lorna Muirhead
President RCM

1st February 1999

Further copies of this report can be obtained from:

The RCOG Bookshop
The Royal College of Obstetricians and Gynaecologists
27 Sussex Place
Regent's Park
London
NW1 4RG

Tel: (0171) 772 6275
Fax: (0171) 724 5991
email: bookshop@rcog.org.uk
website: www.rcog.org.uk

Registered Charity No. 213280

ISBN 1-900364-21-2

Published by the RCOG Press

Contents

Membership

Professor Martin Whittle FRCOG (Chair)
Professor of Fetal Medicine, University of Birmingham
Head of the Academic Department of Obstetrics and Gynaecology

Mrs Belinda Ackerman
Senior Lecturer in Midwifery, Middlesex University, London

Ms Mary Aspinall
Community Midwife, Plymouth Hospital NHS Trust

Miss Rosemary Cranna
Head of Midwifery, Worthing and Southlands Hospital

Mrs Catherine Davis
Midwife, Penrice Materntiy Unit, St Austell, Cornwall

Mr David Davies MRCOG
Consultant Obstetrician and Gynaecologist, St Mary's Hospital, Portsmouth

Ms Frances Day-Stirk
Head of Midwifery Affairs, The Royal College of Midwives

Professor James Drife FRCOG
Professor of Obstetrics and Gynaecology, The General Infirmary, Leeds

Mrs Maggie Elliott
Head of Midwifery, Princess Anne Hospital, Southampton

Mrs Jennifer Kelsall
Midwife, South Manchester University Hospitals NHS Trust

Mrs Michaela Morris
Audit and Clinical Effectiveness Co-ordinator, The Royal College of Midwives

Mrs Lorna Muirhead
President, Royal College of Midwives

Mrs Angela Railton FRCOG
Consultant Obstetrician and Gynaecologist, Hope Hospital, Salford

Professor Stephen Robson MRCOG
Professor of Fetal Medicine, Royal Victoria Infirmary, Newcastle upon Tyne

Professor Charles Rodeck FRCOG
Professor of Obstetrics and Gynaecology, Royal Free and University College Medical School,
University College London

Mr Stephen Walkinshaw MRCOG
Consultant in Maternal and Fetal Medicine, Liverpool Women's Hospital

We acknowledge with thanks advice from the following:

Mrs Beverley Beech
Honorary Secretary, Association for Improvements in the Maternity Services

Ms Meg Goodman
Health Policy Officer, Maternity Alliance

Mr Mark Hackett
Chief Executive, Birmingham Womens' Hospital Trust

Dr Patricia Hamilton FRCP
Consultant in Neonatal Paediatrics, St George's Hospital, London

Dr Antony Rubin FRCA
Consultant Anaesthetist, Magill Department of Anaesthetics, Chelsea & Westminster Hospital

1. Recommendations

1.1 The organisation of labour wards should be reviewed and improved, and if necessary changes implemented to reflect the recommendations in this report.

1.2 All labour wards should have a lead consultant obstetrician and clinical midwife manager.

1.3 The lead obstetrician will be responsible for day to day management, staff deployment, training and support of medical staff. The clinical midwife manager will have parallel responsibilities for midwifery personnel.

1.4 There should be a multidisciplinary labour ward forum comprising, at a minimum, the lead obstetrician, the clinical midwife manager, an obstetric anaesthetist, a neonatal paediatrician, a risk manager, representatives from junior medical and midwifery staff and a consumer representative from the Maternity Services Liaison Committee to review labour ward activity and develop guidelines.

1.5 There should be a set of referenced, evidence-based guidelines which should be dated, signed and reviewed on a regular basis, every one to three years. Past guidelines and protocols should be dated and archived in case they are needed for reference at a later date.

1.6 The documentation and storage of data should be rigorous and precise. The use of computerised documentation, using recognised and acceptable programmes, should be encouraged.

1.7 Staffing, both medical and midwifery, should be in line with the following standards.

▲ At a minimum consultant or equivalent cover should be available in a supervisory capacity for 40 hours during the working week, unless the unit is small and where the majority of women who give birth have had a normal pregnancy.

▲ Junior staffing levels will depend on available training opportunities.

▲ Midwifery staffing levels should be in line with those recommended by the Audit Commission, namely 1.15 midwives per woman in labour.

▲ There should be a clinical midwife leader available on each shift.

1.8 Midwives and medical staff should be able to communicate and consult freely and at an appropriate level.

1.9 The consultant on-call for the labour ward should conduct labour ward rounds at least twice during the day, with a telephone or physical round during the evening.

1.10 In the case of emergencies, anticipated difficult deliveries or whenever a woman's condition gives rise to anxiety, the consultant on the labour ward should be contacted.

1.11 Six monthly multidisciplinary in-service education/training sessions on the management of 'high risk' labours and CTG interpretation should be attended by all clinicians. A log book of attendances should be kept.

1.12 The outcome measures and standards described should be adopted and audited annually in line with best practice.

2. Introduction

2.1 The First Report

The first report from the Royal College of Obstetricians and Gynaecologists on minimum standards of care in labour was published in 1994 [1]. It attempted to establish guidelines for staffing, equipment and general facilities on the labour ward. It sought to identify staffing levels required to provide a safe and effective service. At that time anaesthetists and paediatricians had a much clearer idea of the personnel required than did midwives and obstetricians. The 1994 report emphasised the importance of adequate midwifery staffing, and the need for increased involvement from consultants in terms of supervision and education. No interim survey has been undertaken to assess progress in implementing these suggestions and guidelines.

2.2 Factors contributing to the need for a Second Report

2.2.1 *The Fourth and Fifth Annual Reports of the Confidential Enquiry into Stillbirths and Deaths in Infancy (CESDI)*[2, 3] drew conclusions that gave rise for concern. Over 77% of the intrapartum related deaths identified for study were criticised for sub-optimal care because alternative management 'would reasonably be expected to' have made a difference to outcome in 52% of cases and 'might' have helped in another 25%. 95% of critical comments acknowledged failures in three main areas: to recognise that a problem existed, to take appropriate action, and in communication. "Communication failure" was cited as responsible in 17% of cases with a poor outcome.

The Fourth CESDI Report suggested the problem may lie with working practices, a key issue being the failure of doctors and midwives to work together. The development of a team approach was put forward, so that professionals became familiar with one anothers working practice and worked as a team to provide appropriate care.

The Fifth Report validated the fourth report by reassessing cases using a Second Pass Panel which showed an 80% agreement when significant sub-optimal care was indicated.

2.2.2   *The Confidential Enquiry into Maternal Deaths* 1991-93[4] raised concerns about the possible lack of senior obstetric input into the care of critically ill women and additionally stressed the need for greater involvement of anaesthetists in these cases and for more intensive care facilities. The latest report 1994-96[5] indicates there are still concerns about the failure of consultants to attend and inappropriate delegation of responsibility.

2.2.3   *Changes in Medical Staffing Levels* - Since the first report, the curtailment of junior doctors hours, the New Deal[6], has led to a steady reduction in the availability of junior doctors on the labour ward and to their contribution to service provision. This has important implications for their training and experience. In addition, the experience of Specialist Registrars on completion of training is likely to be less than that of pre-Calman Senior Registrars. As a result consultants are facing an increasing burden for the overall service provision and the anticipated expansion of the consultant grade has not occurred. These two issues, reduced junior doctors hours and increased consultant workload, magnify the problem of inadequate medical staffing of the labour ward.

2.2.4   *Changing Expectations* - In its introductory paragraph, the District Audit report[7] made the following statement:

"With around 700,000 births each year in England and Wales, demand for maternity care is high, costing the Health Service more than £1 billion annually. This study (district audit) is particularly timely due to the recent introduction of government policies aimed at making maternity services more responsive to a woman's needs within available resources. The Department of Health published findings of an expert maternity group in 1993 in a document entitled 'Changing Childbirth'[8]. This policy document has placed maternity services high on the agenda for NHS providers and purchasers.

At the same time as policy initiatives are driving to extend choice, there are concerns about ensuring a safe and efficient service. Patterns of care have changed considerably during the past decade and in particular the effectiveness and desirability of many interventions have been questioned. The dominance of medical models of care is reducing, driven by an increasing recognition of the normality of childbirth".

This has led to an increase in the requirements for midwives and midwifery services. During this time the Government aim, accepted by the Royal College of Obstetricians and Gynaecologists, to establish a consultant based service has developed and with it the expectation that consultants will be more in evidence on the labour ward, involved in the management and decision-making for women whose pregnancies or labours have become complicated.

2.2.5   *Medical Litigation* - The NHS Litigation Authority gives a figure of £242,782,343 as the total claims paid out for obstetrics since 1 April 1995, 64% of claims in all specialties. This does not take into consideration the human cost, nor the valuable time spent by hospital personnel investigating complaints. The very large increase in medical litigation has much to do with labour ward activity. Cases are particularly vulnerable when there is an apparent lack of consultant involvement in the management of complicated labour and complex obstetric problems.

2.2.6   *Low Morale* - Some labour wards are excessively busy, with too few staff and, in certain circumstances, inadequate equipment. Difficulties appear to arise because staff fail to recognise the warning signs of impending clinical problems. This phenomenon of denial can arise not only from inadequate training and supervision, but also fatigue, stress and an insidious increase in work activity. Low morale may result from weak or inadequate leadership and improvements would be expected if stronger direction were provided by the clinical midwife manager and lead consultant together. Low morale can be exacerbated by staff shortages. A recent survey has highlighted the lowest number of practising midwives for a decade[9]. The NHS Executive letter EL(95)77 recommends a minimum of F grade for all midwives. Significant improvements in recruitment and retention have been noted in units that have implemented this recommendation.

3.   Organisation

3.1   General Principles

3.1.1   A good working relationship between the multi-disciplinary team - midwives, medical, ancillary, managerial staff - and the women in their care is crucial to ensure optimal birth outcomes. This requires an organisational structure for both midwives and medical staff with explicit lines of communication. Each Trust should have a clinical midwife manager who has overall responsibility for the management of the Labour Ward, a named midwife shift co-ordinator and a clinical midwife leader who is there to give advice and support or to resource other midwives. There should be a lead consultant with specific responsibility for obstetric aspects of the labour ward.

3.1.2   A number of key professionals are needed to address the quality aspects of service delivery including guideline development, setting and monitoring of standards, and other organisational issues. Whilst team working is essential if women are to receive optimum care, it is also recognised that a midwife is professionally accountable for the care she gives and that another professional cannot be held accountable for any acts or omissions on her part unless they have had involvement in that care. Such involvement should be clearly documented, the areas of responsibility between doctors and midwives clearly defined and recorded to ensure clarity. The lead professional should be identified on the case notes and where this is the midwife, the consultant obstetrician's name should not be recorded on the notes.

3.1.3 The main organisational drive should come from a Labour Ward Forum. As a minimum this should comprise the lead obstetrician, the clinical midwife manager, an obstetric anaesthetist, a neonatal paediatrician, a risk manager, representatives from junior medical and midwifery staff, and a consumer representative from the Maternity Services Liaison Committee.

3.1.4 The Forum should formalise an explicit system which ensures women receive the care appropriate to their needs. Thus midwives will be responsible for women in normal labour whilst women with complicated labours or with complex obstetric problems will be looked after by a combination of midwives and medical staff.

3.2 Risk Management

3.2.1 *Clinical Negligence Scheme for Trusts (CNST)* - The CNST has identified the importance of consultant input to the labour ward, and suggests that a standard of at least 40 hours of consultant sessions during the working week on the labour ward is desirable. It has identified a number of standards applicable to the labour ward (Appendix 1).

3.2.2 *Documentation* - It has become crucial, not only for medico-legal purposes but also for good clinical practice, to have in place systems to document and record clinical decisions and events. The archiving of all data, including out of date protocols, is absolutely vital. The careful storage of cardiotocographs, partograms and anaesthetic records should be mandatory. One individual, perhaps the risk manager, should be responsible for ensuring appropriate methods are adopted.

It is also important for practitioners to keep contemporary notes and accurately document events - date and time, printed name and signature, written in black ink[10]. Appropriate abbreviations may only be used once the terminology has been written in full with the relevant abbreviation adjacent to it. The first indicator of success in Changing Childbirth[8] recommends that all women be entitled to carry their own notes.

3.2.3 *Communication* - Adequate facilities for communicating with non-English speakers is an essential component of good care which may help to minimise potential cases of litigation. Interpreting/advocacy workers should be available on a 24-hour basis and the individual woman's needs should be identified in the antenatal period. The practice of courteous introduction and clear staff identification is recommended.

3.2.4   *Security* - This is an issue of increasing importance for staff, mothers and babies. A robust system must be in place for their protection . An effective system of staff identification and strict criteria for the labelling and security for the newborn infant are essential[11].

3.2.5   *Transfer from Primary Care Settings* - On occasion the need for women to transfer to an acute hospital setting will occur. This report endorses the recommended transfer arrangements quoted in the CESDI Fifth Report[3]. "Arrangements for transfer to hospital should be made at the earliest indication, by whichever professional is present. Where a midwife feels transfer is needed and the woman agrees, this should be done as soon as possible. Waiting, for example, for the GP to arrive and confirm the decision is rarely appropriate. Hospital staff must be forewarned of the transfer and the reasons for it. Staff of appropriate specialty and seniority should be available to meet the woman/baby in order to assess the situation and decide on further management".

4. Staffing Levels

4.1   Midwives

4.1.1   The need to review midwifery labour ward staffing is discussed in the recent Audit Commission Report "First Class Delivery"[12]. The Audit Commission confirms a good practice standard of 1.15 midwives to one woman in labour and discusses organisation of staff. This level of staffing should be achieved on at least 60% of occasions. It states "Trusts can take several steps to improve the flexibility of labour ward staffing overall and the provision of support staff, and how staff are deployed in response to workload, taking into account the case mix as well as peaks and troughs in activity".

4.1.2   An important factor which will affect labour ward staffing is the need for midwives to assist in the operating theatre. In some units midwives have traditionally been involved with scrubbing for caesarean sections. They are also required to receive the baby at delivery and assist the paediatrician whenever necessary. In many units midwives are responsible for the immediate post-operative care and recovery of the mother and baby within the operating theatre prior to transfer to the ward. This will have staffing implications.

4.1.3 The presence of an intensive care or high dependency unit within the confines of the delivery unit will also have a bearing on the number of midwives required. These calculations should be made at a local level, again dependent on workload and casemix. It is possible, for example, that a particular unit with a high dependency room may use that room very infrequently making it unnecessary to provide more midwives on that basis alone.

4.1.4 Provision of "continuous care of mother and fetus for the duration of an epidural blockade" is imperative. In units where the ratio of one to one midwife to woman standard cannot be met "epidural blockade should not be instituted"[13].

4.1.5 The number of midwives required to provide care on any particular labour ward will be dependent upon local workload activity in conjunction with casemix and pattern of service provision (see 3.1.1). Various workload analysis tools such as Telford, Aberdeen and Birthrate[14] have been developed. The RCM recommends the use of Birthrate as a workload dependency and skill mix tool (see Appendix 2).

4.1.6 The above are minimum midwife staffing requirements. Additional staff will be required to ensure the availability of a second midwife when required, for example to staff the operating theatre.

4.2 Obstetric Staff

4.2.1 The Central Negligence Scheme for Trusts' proposed standard (see Appendix 1) of at least 40 hours of consultant time during the working week on the labour ward is considered by the Working Party to be an appropriate level of cover. Staff involved in labour ward activity are identified in Figure 1. Career grade doctors adequately qualified to staff the labour ward at a senior level may also be used in the organisation.

4.2.2 It is seen from Figure 2 that there are various categories of cover from on-call through to full cover. These suggestions are dependent on the workload and complexity of work and they are for guidance only. However, these suggestions are the bare minimum that are required for adequate cover. The categories apply to consultant units and not midwifery-led units.

Figure 1 **Medical Staffing**

Title	Definition
Consultant	Specialist holding an NHS contract
Trainee	Specialist Registrar (SpR)- Senior (years 4/5) Junior (years 1-3)
Senior House Officer (SHO)	Pre SpR graduate. SHOs may have MRCOG but varying experience. Could act-up if appropriately experienced.

Figure 2   **Definitions of Level of Cover for Consultants**

Available	Minimum would be consultant ward round early and late to identify and assess problems. Available within the hospital, but may have other commitments. There should be at least two set consultant sessions a week.
	Out of hours On-call (1800-0800 hours and at weekends). The consultant must be available for the labour ward within 30 minutes. At weekends a daily labour ward round and either a physical or telephone round in the evening is required, which would increase commensurate with workload.
Supervisory	Set consultant sessions on the labour ward; target is 40 hours/week Monday to Friday. The consultant's work plan will indicate no other commitment during the labour ward session.
	Out of hours On-call (1800-0800 hours and at weekends). The consultant must be available for the labour ward within 30 minutes. At weekends a daily labour ward round and either a physical or telephone round in the evening is required, which would increase commensurate with workload.
Full cover	This entails 24 hour consultant involvement in the labour ward with no other commitment. This should be the aim of all units delivering over 6000 babies/year in the first instance, moving to 4000 in tertiary referral centres in the future.

Figure 3 **Staff Cover required for different categories of consultant units**

Category	Definition	Consultant	Trainee
A	Units delivering <1000 per year, small, essentially low risk units	Available	SHO
B	Units delivering 1000 - 4000 babies per year	Supervisory	Specialist Registrar + SHO
C	Units delivering > 4000 babies per year and/or tertiary referrals	Full cover *or* Supervisory	SpR (years 4/5) and/or SpR (years 1-3) SHO

4.2.3   Figure 3 indicates staff deployment based on workload. The workload cut-offs are arbitrary and Figure 3 should be seen as the framework for local interpretation. The terms low and high risk relate to referral patterns; a unit delivering a low number of babies overall but with many high risk cases would see itself in a higher category than A.

4.2.4   It is vital that consultants and their Trusts do not see these labour ward activities as <u>additional</u> roles. They must form part of the consultant's agreed job plan. Changes are likely to have considerable implications for the overall cost of the service, and if implemented will require an expansion of consultant numbers.

4.2.5 In Figure 3, for Category A there should be a consultant plus one member of junior staff who should have at least 12 months' experience in obstetrics and gynaecology. Even in this model one or more of the senior staff should have some specific organisational responsibility for the labour ward. Whether the junior doctor post should be recognised for training, ie a Specialist Registrar post, would be for local discussion.

4.2.6 A Category B unit would require a consultant in the labour ward for 40 hours per week. Their role would be to supervise and educate trainees and to audit activity with daily reviews. One or more consultants should develop a major supervisory role in medical management, a responsibility which might rotate amongst the consultant body. It is not envisaged that the consultant will act in isolation, and the notion that they may replace the SpRs is not acceptable. Units in categories B and C, which constitute the majority of those in the National Health Service (NHS), will have a very significant training role for both doctors and midwives.

4.2.7 Labour ward activity continues 24 hours a day, 7 days a week. When on-call out of hours (1800-0800 hrs) and at weekends consultants must be available at all times within 30 minutes. At weekends, depending on workload, a minimum requirement would be a daily labour ward round and either a telephone call or physical ward round in the evening. In busy units the frequency of ward rounds would need to be increased.

4.2.8 Category C provides for the busiest and highest risk care. Consideration of 24 hour consultant cover means that the running of these services will have considerable resource implications. The presence of senior cover at this level can only be justified by the need to care for considerable numbers of high risk cases. A lead consultant will be responsible for overall medical organisation of the department. The consultant of the day will usually be backed by one or two specialist registrars and one senior house officer. These units will have an important responsibility in both basic and advanced training in high risk obstetric practice and the extent of junior cover will depend on workload and training opportunities.

4.2.9 Currently four units in the UK deliver more than 6000 babies a year, although this may change as pressures from neonatal unit staffing problems and other essential resources become stretched, leading to the amalgamation of smaller units. Such units may justify full cover. These large units may feel that the extra investment in more consultants to provide such cover would be worthwhile and they could act as pilot units for such a scheme. However, it is essential that no unit moves to the level of full consultant cover until staffing levels are deemed adequate.

4.2.10 A 24 hour consultant based service has major implications for consultants in terms of job plans, remuneration, living-in facilities and time off duty. Since consultants who devote much of their time to the labour ward may do little or no gynaecology, their future career development needs careful consideration. This will need to be addressed as part of the annual job plan and the personal development plans as suggested in A First Class Service [15].

4.3 Anaesthetists

4.3.1 At least one consultant anaesthetist should have a major interest in obstetric anaesthesia and intensive care of the pregnant woman and devote a large part of the working week to obstetrics. This consultant anaesthetist should have overall responsibility for managing the anaesthetic service. It is estimated that there should be one consultant (notional half day) to 500 deliveries up to 3000, and full cover above that number to assist in teaching the trainees and providing support for them. If the changes in staffing envisaged for obstetricians occur in anaesthetics and the service becomes consultant-based an increase in numbers would be necessary. The Obstetric Anaesthetists Association have recommended minimum standards for obstetric anaesthesia services[13].

4.3.2 Anaesthetic cover must be immediately available throughout 24 hours and the anaesthetist involved must have more than one year of experience in anaesthesia, and have access to prompt advice and support from more senior anaesthetic colleagues. Trainees must be of sufficient numbers to allow them to gain supervised clinical experience, to attend teaching sessions and to take part in rotas permitting legal hours of work under current guidelines.

4.3.3 Women should have available an epidural pain relief service and both regional and general anaesthesia for operative delivery. The anaesthetic response time should be such that a caesarean section can be started within 30 minutes of the clinical decision to proceed.

4.3.4 A dedicated anaesthetic assistant should be available at all times. This may be an operating department practitioner (ODP) or registered nurse who has completed the English National Board (ENB) 182 course in anaesthesia or equivalent[16].

4.3.5 Anaesthetic advice should be available for women attending an antenatal clinic. For example, when problems have arisen in a previous labour many women have anxieties that can often be allayed by an appropriate consultation. Information concerning analgesia and anaesthesia should be available to all through parenthood education or by written information.

4.3.6　All women requiring conduction or general anaesthesia should be visited by an anaesthetist both before and after the procedure.

4.4　Paediatricians

4.4.1　Minimum standards with respect to the immediate care of the newborn require that basic resuscitation skills should be available wherever a baby is born, be it in hospital or at home. The failure to provide this basic support is likely to result in a potentially unfavourable outcome and will fall below acceptable standards of care.

4.4.2　It is more difficult to calculate paediatric requirements per 1000 deliveries since the numbers of staff needed relate more to the numbers of intensive care cots in the neonatal unit than to the numbers of births in the delivery unit. Nevertheless it is possible to define certain standards.

4.4.3　For a delivery unit to which there are no, or few, *in utero* or *ex utero* transfers, the basic requirements is at least one consultant paediatrician available on-call. This person would usually be one of two or three consultant paediatricians, one having a special interest in the newborn. Junior paediatric staff should be available twenty-four hours a day to cover both general paediatric and neonatal duties on the same site. There should be a professional immediately available at all times who can provide advanced neonatal resuscitation including endotracheal intubation[17].

4.4.4　Referral from other centres is likely to have a greater impact on the paediatric service than on the obstetric service. When there is a substantial *in utero* transfer policy there should be one consultant paediatrician on-call from a team of three, at least one of whom would be an accredited neonatologist. The middle grade paediatric staff, who should be resident, would be available at all times and should have no other commitments outside the maternity hospital or neonatal unit. Resident SHOs in the unit would provide 24 hour cover.

4.4.5　In small hospitals without a paediatric service it will be essential that all medical and midwifery staff are appropriately trained in neonatal resuscitation[18]. This should be an absolute requirement for such units.

4.5　General Medical Cover

During labour women with medical problems such as diabetes, heart disease, severe anaemia or sickle cell disease should have access to a general physician with particular interest in pregnancy and their medical condition. Where no such physician is available guidelines should exist for the management of medical disorders. Clear arrangements should be made to ensure adequate cover at all times. In complex cases a clear management plan, indicating the relevant personnel to be involved, should be displayed in the notes.

4.6 Ancillary Help

It is essential that there is adequate ancillary help on the delivery unit. In particular there should be a ward clerk or receptionist available 24 hours a day unless labour ward activity is very low. Some secretarial support may also be necessary. There should be an adequate number of maternity care assistants and domestic service staff to provide basic and yet vital services to women, their families and labour companions.

5. Staffing Roles

5.1 Midwives

5.1.1   In the 1998 Midwives Rules and Code of Practice[19] Rule 40 states that "in an emergency or where a deviation from the norm which is outside her current sphere of practice becomes apparent in the mother or baby during the antenatal, intranatal or postnatal periods, a practising midwife shall call to her assistance a registered medical practitioner or such other qualified health professional as has the requisite skills and experience". This means that the midwife's first consultation may be with an appropriately experienced midwife colleague.

5.1.2   In addition to being mentors for student midwives, midwives have an increasing role in teaching and mentoring junior doctors and when appropriate medical students. In order to accommodate this extension to their role, it is essential that there is an increase in midwifery establishment.

5.1.3   It is recognised that, regardless of the place of birth, the majority of women will be cared for by midwives. There is agreement that the midwife plays a central role in the care of women in labour. The minimum standard is that each woman should have one midwife with her throughout labour, preferably one who she knows. It is the unanimous view that one midwife to one woman should be the standard. There is clear evidence that the provision of continuous skilled support not only enhances maternal satisfaction with labour but also reduces the need for a wide range of medical interventions.[7,12,20,21]

5.1.4   Midwives have responsibility for the care and management of women in normal labour when they work as autonomous practitioners. In the care of women with complex pregnancies they work as partners with obstetricians, anaesthetists and paediatricians to ensure a satisfactory outcome for mothers and babies. If women develop complications during the course of their labour, the need for flexibility and good communication in the management of the labour is essential.

5.1.5 The role of the midwife is to recognise complications if they arise, for example, lack of progress in labour, or a problem with the fetus detected most often by monitoring the fetal condition. If complications do arise, midwives are able to respond within a multi-disciplinary team[18]. Midwives should work within a professional environment which acknowledges and fosters the inter-related and complementary responsibilities of each practitioner. Such mutual respect should enhance care but it must be based on agreed standards to ensure effective communication and co-operation[22].

5.1.6 In larger units, especially those concerned with the management of high risk labour, there needs to be a core of midwives whose major role is to provide care for women with complications or who are critically ill. These midwives will require additional skills concerned with the management of complex obstetric problems[23]. The number of such midwives required will depend on the number of high dependency women. We would recommend that there should be at least one midwife with high dependency skills per room per shift, or as many as are appropriate for individual units.

5.2 Junior Medical Staff

5.2.1 Traditionally, junior medical staff have provided the main medical input to the running of the labour ward. It is the time when clinicians start to develop their organisational ability and undertake decision-making and operative work. It is an exciting and interesting time for junior obstetricians. To do the job well requires hard work, a good deal of concentration and an ability to work under stressful situations. Increasing patient demands and rising levels of litigation have increased the stresses on junior staff.

5.2.2 The challenge is to find ways of providing junior staff with training, without detracting from the service provision.

5.2.3 The shorter working hours of junior medical staff have led to a number of problems. The shift system itself can lead to fragmentation of patient care, although with proper organisation this can be minimised. One mechanism for improving continuity at the change over of medical staff is the principle of a "baton bleep" which is handed from one doctor to the next on-call.

5.2.4 A medical team has its own hierarchy, from SHO to consultant. As with all effective teams, each member must have a clear idea about their own role, with a clear chain of command. The composition of these teams, with regard to individual training needs and skill mix, would be the responsibility of the lead consultant for the labour ward.

5.2.5   Junior staff grades are divided into senior house officers (SHOs) (who may be GP trainees) and Specialist Registrars (SpRs) subdivided into years 1 to 3 and years 4/5 [Figure 1]. It should be recognised that most SHOs will have little or no previous experience in obstetrics. The individual's level of experience needs to be taken into account when organising service cover. Inexperienced SHOs are likely to get their best instruction from midwife colleagues. They will need to learn the basic skills of labour ward management. They should not be placed in a position of providing service support on the labour ward unless appropriately experienced as judged from their personal log book.

5.2.6   SpRs in years 1 to 3 should have sufficient experience and training to undertake some operative deliveries and to perform basic decision-making on the labour ward. In general it would not be appropriate for them to undertake the training of SHOs since they themselves would only have a basic level of knowledge. Under certain circumstances the SpR in years 1 to 3 may be considerably experienced, in which case they could be given additional responsibility.

5.2.7   An SpR in years 4/5 should be capable of undertaking most operative procedures on the labour ward and performing routine decision-making. They will relate to and consult closely with the consultant in charge. Responsibility for the day to day running of a labour ward has always been regarded as a crucial part of the training for SpRs in years 4/5. It is usually the first time that they will have the opportunity to initiate decision-making for more major clinical matters and it is essential that they have the opportunity to discuss issues and to learn from the consultant on-call for the day. This balance between over-supervision by the consultant and the chance for the SpR in years 4/5 to initiate their own decisions is a fine one. In the case of emergency abdominal deliveries when difficulties with delivery are anticipated, or when there is anxiety about a patient's condition, the consultant on-call should be contacted and be available within 30 minutes.

5.3   Consultants

5.3.1   The consultant role on the labour ward has often been seen as one of providing cover rather than of active involvement. The reduction in junior doctors hours resulting from the New Deal highlighted the need for increasing consultant activity. Hitherto the consultant role was ill-defined, but a number of key activities, familiar in other areas of consultant-based activity, are also applicable to the labour ward.

All consultants who work on the labour ward should:

    a) provide clinical leadership and lead by example

    b) train and educate staff in a multidisciplinary team

    c) ensure effective teamwork

    d) develop and implement standards of obstetric practice

    e) bring experience to clinical diagnosis and opinion

    f) audit the effectiveness of practice and modify it as required.

5.3.2   The concept of a lead obstetrician on the labour ward is important. Every Trust should identify a consultant to fulfil this role or arrange another model that achieves the same aim. This person, in conjunction with a clinical midwife manager, would have overall responsibility for the organisation, standard setting and audit on the labour ward.

5.3.3   Labour ward activity must form an identified component of the consultant obstetrician's job plan. Figure 3 provides suggested levels of cover for consultants dependent on local circumstances. These standards may already exist in many Trusts; where they are not met Trusts should move towards achieving them as quickly as possible.

5.3.4   Although no definitive evidence exists which links the presence of consultants on the labour ward with improvements in outcome, it seems reasonable to conclude that greater consultant involvement will lead to better organisation and enhanced clinical decision-making. This should contribute to a reduction in the numbers of intrapartum deaths and asphyxiated babies[2] and in maternal deaths[4]. In addition, there may be fewer, but more appropriate, inductions and better management of labour, perhaps reducing the need for caesarean sections. A recent survey[24] showed, for example, particularly in primigravida, that more careful assessment in labour with more liberal use of fetal blood sampling might well reduce caesarean section rates. Further, in a study from Wales[25], it was suggested that intrapartum complications occurred more commonly at night and during traditional holiday periods, the implication being that at these times less experienced advice was available.

5.3.5   The above data, whilst not conclusively indicating the potential impact of more consultant involvement on the labour ward, are suggestive. Clearly further research needs to be done in this area. Whether or not evidence of benefit exists, the fact remains that a consultant presence is being increasingly required because of the issues identified in 2.2.

6. Training, Accreditation and Continuing Education

6.1 Midwives

An important quality issue is the maintenance of skills. It is a responsibility of individual midwives to make sure their skills are up to date [19] in line with the PREP (Post Registration Education and Practice) requirements, and annual interviews with the named supervisor will facilitate this development[26].

6.2 Junior Medical Staff

6.2.1   The training objectives of junior doctors are set out in the basic and main log books they use. Acquisition of practical skills can be difficult with the reduction in working hours. In addition to learning new skills, junior staff need to maintain those already acquired. A series of programmes for updating junior staff in cardiotocography (CTG), partograms and manual dexterity on the labour ward must be available. It is important to achieve an appropriate balance between new learning and the maintenance of former skills. Consultants will have a major responsibility to ensure that relevant staff attend and gain the necessary knowledge.

6.2.2   *Accreditation* - Junior staff now have an accreditation process which runs through the Calman training programme.

6.3 Consultants

6.3.1   Some consultants fear they do not now have sufficient skills to undertake labour ward activity. Regular updating of skills and feedback from specific labour incidents should be seen as part of continuing professional development (CPD). It should not be assumed that consultants, even though they may have done many years of labour ward activity as senior registrars, will necessarily be comfortable to go back there without updating their skills. An internal programme of CPD, to include the reading of CTGs and management problems, particularly as they relate to the seriously sick patient, should ensure that labour ward skills are maintained. This would have cost implications.

6.3.2   *Accreditation* - The process of CPD goes some way towards personal accreditation. There is however an argument for separate labour ward accreditation. Evaluation and monitoring of standards of care in labour wards is something which both the RCOG and RCM need to consider. The process of accreditation would be better arranged by the specialty rather than by an outside agency. Nevertheless, as identified by the General Medical Council, regular updating and maintenance of standards are essential features of being a doctor [27].

7. Developing Standards

7.1   Each Trust should develop an evidence-based course in the early detection of the compromised fetus incorporating fetal monitoring, intermittent auscultation and CTG presentation. This should be supported by relevant literature, eg the Crimson file[28], available on the ward.

7.2   It is important to develop critical incident analysis, de-briefing and regular multidisciplinary labour ward meetings (case review and associated CTG interpretation). All these will provide ready opportunity for constructive, objective dialogue.

7.3   The CESDI study identified CTG interpretation as a major area of weakness. There should be regular joint CTG and weekly case review meetings for both doctors and midwives. A log of attendance should be kept.

Standard 1   Evidence of staff attendance at weekly multidisciplinary labour ward meetings, case review, partogram discussion and associated CTG interpretation.

7.4   The pro-active approach to group training, including regular assessment of knowledge, is a vital component to ensure that team function is up to date and clinically effective. Individual case management review develops a conducive learning environment and promotes multidisciplinary communication. Interaction of this nature may improve the team's response to any problems that arise.

Standard 2   Evidence of ongoing multi-professional education programmes and availability of reference texts.

7.5   Each Trust should provide a multidisciplinary forum including consumer groups to exchange views and develop agreed guidance for best practice. Guidelines should be evidence-based and reviewed annually.

Standard 3   Evidence of monthly forum programme, recorded attendance and annual activity review.

7.6   The adoption of three monthly obstetric emergency "practice runs", comprising decision to delivery interval, patient collapse and major haemorrhage, is to be encouraged.

Standard 4   Each Trust should provide auditable evidence of three monthly 'ad hoc' practice runs.

7.7   Critical incident analysis is an effective educational and management tool and its use should be incorporated into the philosophy and daily management of labour wards.

Standard 5   Each Trust should demonstrate evidence of its mechanism and application.

7.8 Facilities should exist on, or adjacent to, the labour ward to provide information technology systems (CD-ROM) giving access to current evidence-based information. Training should be available.

Standard 6 Each Trust should provide well equipped resources and facilities for on site learning.

7.9 The following outcome measures should be recorded and reviewed quarterly with an annual summary review:

Inductions - indications and outcomes
Augmentation of labour
Percentage of labours lasting longer than 18 hours
Episiotomy rates
Epidural rates
Total deliveries
Elective caesarean section rates and indications
Emergency caesarean sections - incidence and indications
Instrumental delivery rates - ventouse, forceps
Intrapartum stillbirths
Apgar scores less than 7 at 5 minutes
Need for neonatal resuscitation
Admissions to special care for babies weighing more than 2.5 kg
Incidence of primary postpartum haemorrhage
% of complicated deliveries attended by a consultant
Breast feeding rates

Standard 7 Each Trust should collect and review the above statistics, identifying trends and any intervention.

7.10 The following labour ward staffing levels should be recorded and reviewed quarterly with an annual summary review.

(a) **Midwifery staffing** should be sufficient

    i) to provide a ratio of 1.15:1 midwife to woman in normal labour

    ii) to ensure an experienced midwife (clinical leader) is available for each shift

(b) **Obstetric staff**

    i) A doctor of at least 12 months' experience should be resident on labour ward or available within 5 minutes

    ii) A doctor of at least 3 years' obstetric experience should be available within 30 minutes

(c) **Anaesthetic staff**

    i) An anaesthetist with at least one year's experience should be available within 10 minutes

    ii) The maximum response time from decision to start of an emergency caesarean section should be 30 minutes

iii) All women requiring conduction or general anaesthesia should be visited by an anaesthetist before an elective procedure

iv) Over 80% of women having a caesarean section should be offered a regional block

v) A named consultant should be responsible for ensuring standards for obstetric analgesia and resuscitation

vi) Staff should be "drilled" in managing acute obstetric emergencies

Standard 8 Each Trust should demonstrate evidence of collection and review of the above staffing statistics.

7.11 The labour ward consultant on-call should conduct a ward round at least twice during the day, with a telephone or physical round during the evening.

7.12 There should be a minimum of 40 hours consultant supervision for labour wards, unless the unit is low risk and delivers less than 1000 babies per year.

7.13 A consultant should be present at, or on the delivery suite for, at least 10% of complicated deliveries, such as caesarean section.

Standard 9 Each Trust should demonstrate documented evidence eg labour ward log book signed, with date and time, by the attending consultant.

7.14 Labour ward facilities should provide a safe, homely and private environment. Special facilities for bereaved parents should be available.

Standard 10 Each Trust should provide facilities as described within the next 5 years.

7.15 A comprehensive list of auditable standards is enclosed as Appendix 4.

8. Facilities and Equipment

8.1 The Delivery Rooms

8.1.1 While a pleasant environment is an important element in creating the right atmosphere, it is the attitude of staff which is of greater value. All personnel on the labour ward should work towards creating a pleasant and relaxed atmosphere in which couples can share in the experience of childbirth.

8.1.2 Some units have been able to create a room which is welcoming and homely but at the same time provides facilities to undertake anything from normal delivery to caesarean section. This might be difficult to achieve in many current labour wards, but should be an aim for the future. Planning should include representatives of consumer groups.

8.1.3 The delivery rooms should be decorated and arranged to make the physical environment more pleasant and less clinical and threatening for childbirth. All units should be subjected to an access survey by a disability group in order to ensure requirements of the Disability Discrimination Act[29].

8.1.4 The furniture in the delivery unit should be comfortable for the woman and allow her to adopt a variety of positions during labour, as well as being adaptable for both normal and operative vaginal delivery.

8.1.5 Facilities should be available to accommodate bereaved parents, preferably so that all their care can be given in a separate room, from which they can be discharged.

8.1.6 The working party is unanimous in its belief that every effort must be made to improve the experience of childbirth in hospital whilst maintaining maximum safety. Privacy for the woman and her partner should be respected by keeping interruptions and unnecessary access to the delivery rooms to the minimum.

8.2 Intensive Care and High Dependency Units

8.2.1 Prompt access to a high dependency unit, intensive care unit and/or resuscitation facilities must be available. The extent to which these facilities are made available will depend on the workload, case-mix and the local circumstances.

8.2.2 As part of obstetric practice women will occasionally develop serious problems with major organ failure, clotting disorders and severe haemorrhage. All units should be able to provide some level of resuscitation or high dependency care including cardiovascular monitoring, pulse oximetry, rapid transfusions of fluids or blood and ventilation, for up to 6 hours, whilst awaiting transfer to an intensive care unit. The high dependency unit may be a recovery room or a separate, dedicated area. Appropriately skilled midwifery and medical staff should be available, together with all the necessary monitoring equipment including oximeters, capnographs and devices for measuring direct vascular pressure. The same documentation (ie charts, etc) as used for standard intensive care units should be utilised.

8.2.3 The demand for such units will depend on case-mix and referral patterns. Nevertheless provision should probably be made for up to ten high dependency cases per thousand deliveries per year. It has been reported that about one ITU admission will arise per 1000 deliveries [30]. There should be recognised routes of access to intensive care units in the same or other hospitals, together with equipment and personnel for safe transfer. Arrangements must be in place for small units having to transfer women requiring intensive care to another hospital.

8.2.4 *Midwifery staffing* - As far as midwifery cover for such units is concerned, it will be necessary to develop a cadre of midwives who have particular experience and expertise in the management of the critically ill woman. These midwives will be part of the midwifery establishment and will require special training in intensive care and should be allotted time to attend regular updating courses[22].

8.2.5 *Medical Staff* - When a medical opinion is required, cover should ensure that women are not kept waiting longer than 30 minutes and that the doctor is of adequate seniority to ensure that appropriate decisions about onward care are taken. There should be clear guidelines for junior staff concerning subsequent management.

8.3 Theatre

Operating theatres dedicated for obstetrics should be close to the delivery unit or preferably in it. It is felt that one theatre is sufficient for a delivery load of up to 4000 babies a year. A delivery rate above this would require two operating theatres so that simultaneous procedures could be performed. Larger units would also benefit from a second theatre to handle infected cases, i.e. hepatitis, HIV and sepsis. In most units one of the delivery rooms can serve as a "back-up" operating theatre under extreme circumstances. All delivery rooms should have available suction equipment, oxygen and, if appropriate, anaesthetic gases. All equipment must be appropriately maintained to ensure safe and effective function.

8.4 Laboratory Facilities

8.4.1 It is essential that wherever women are being delivered in hospital there should be adequate laboratory facilities, if not on-site then within easy reach. Of particular importance is the availability of blood and blood products in case of major haemorrhage. Out of hours staffing may be difficult for many laboratories but it is essential that at least cross-matching services and blood clotting screens are readily available. It is advisable that O Rh negative blood should be immediately available and that cross-matched blood should be available to the clinician within forty-five minutes of the sample being drawn from the woman. Biochemistry facilities are also important and results of tests should be available to the clinician within $1^{1}/_{2}$ to 2 hours of the blood sample being drawn. Tests which will be undertaken on an emergency basis should be agreed between the biochemistry department and clinicians.

8.4.2 If possible there should be facilities for Gram staining and microscopic examination of specimens such as urine and amniotic fluid; microbiological culture should be available on a 24 hour basis.

8.5 Fetal Heart Rate Monitors

Fetal heart rate monitoring forms an essential part of intrapartum care of women in high risk labour. The numbers of monitors required will depend on workload and case-mix; units dealing with high risk cases would need a greater number. Between 2 to 4 fetal heart rate monitors per 1000 deliveries a year is considered appropriate. This should include at least one instrument capable of monitoring twins. Traditional auscultation together with intermittent fetal heart monitoring (using a cardiotocograph) is the recommended method of fetal assessment in many units. Clear guidelines to help identify cases suitable for continuous fetal heart monitoring should be established in light of evidence which suggests that "continuous fetal heart monitoring increases the likelihood of subsequent operative delivery independently of other factors"[31].

8.6 Blood Gas and pH Analysers

The ability to assess fetal blood gases by modern, easily-used equipment should be available in any unit undertaking continuous fetal heart rate monitoring. The two should not be separated. Ideally the blood gas analyser should be able to measure pH, pO_2, pCO_2. The routine measurement of cord blood gases is essential for all caesarean sections or instrumental deliveries for fetal distress indication, and consideration should be given to measurement of cord blood gases following all deliveries. The presence of normal gases, but not pH alone, largely excludes hypoxia as a cause of brain damage and would have important medico-legal implications. This policy also has an educational role.

8.7 Ultrasound Equipment

An ultrasound scanner should be available on the labour ward. This equipment should be capable of producing a good image and reliable measurements. An ultrasound examination during labour can be of vital importance, particularly for confirmation of presentation in the obese, in women who are bleeding and when there are concerns about fetal condition. This equipment may be used by both medical and midwifery staff, but only when personnel are appropriately trained. All ultrasound equipment should comply with EEC/IEC/157 directives.

8.8 Anaesthetic and Resuscitation Equipment

Operating theatres, anaesthetic rooms and recovery rooms should contain equipment to recognised standards for anaesthesia, monitoring and resuscitation[17]. Anaesthesia should only be administered when there is an oxygen analyser (with alarms) available and devices to enable leaks, disconnections, re-breathing or over-pressure to be detected. Continuous monitoring of ventilation and cardiovascular status is essential. Minimal monitoring should include a pulse oximeter, electrocardiogram and capnograph and non-invasive blood pressure measurement. The ability to measure intravascular pressures and body temperature should be available together with peripheral nerve stimulation when neuromuscular blocking agents are administered. The use of emergency resuscitation equipment and cardiac arrest procedures should be displayed and visible to all. There should be regular training and refresher courses for all staff on at least an annual basis[18].

8.9   Intravenous Therapy

Intravenous therapy should be provided through a range of syringe pumps and infusion systems, all in good working order.

8.10   Neonatal Resuscitation Equipment

The Royal College of Paediatrics and Child Health makes recommendations for equipment for resuscitation at home and in a hospital[32] (see Appendix 3).

9. Conclusions

9.1   Concerns from CESDI and the Confidential Enquiry into Maternal Deaths have indicated the need for a fresh look at the organisation of labour wards. This document seeks to establish benchmarks for the provision of a standard of care which will offer a safe and pleasant childbirth experience.

9.2   This report, in addressing issues relating to organisation of labour wards, acknowledges:

▲   the increased involvement from consultants on the labour ward in the care of women with complex or complicated pregnancies and in the supervision and education of medical staff

▲   the central role of midwives as autonomous practitioners of the norm, together with their role as partners with obstetricians, anaesthetists and paediatricians in the care of women with complex and complicated labours.

9.3   Changes in medical staffing at junior level and demand for increasing consultant involvement in the labour ward, greater focus on woman-centred care, an extension to the midwife's teaching role, recruitment and retention crises in midwifery staffing have serious implications for the service[18,8,33].

9.4   It is important to try to match resources and facilities with workload. The document outlines minimum staffing requirements for midwives and doctors. Additional staff over and above this will be needed in specific situations, eg midwifery staff in the operating theatre.

9.5   This report provides healthcare planners, unit managers and clinical directors with guidelines on which to base realistic costing of this particular service. Certain quality and clinical effectiveness issues have been identified, which include supervision (statutory and clinical) as well as basic and continuing training of all staff. Each hospital will need to adapt the model suggested to achieve the standards in their own circumstances.

9.6 Where deliveries occur outside the hospital environment, it is essential that there is a robust plan with clear guidelines about transfer arrangements should problems arise.

10. References

1. Report of the RCOG Working Party on Minimum Standards of Care in Labour (1994). RCOG, London.

2. Confidential Enquiry into Stillbirths and Deaths in Infancy Fourth Annual Report, 1 January - 31 December 1995 (1997). Maternal and Child Health Research Consortium, 188 Baker Street, London.

3. Confidential Enquiry into Stillbirths and Deaths in Infancy Fifth Annual Report, 1 January - 31 December 1996 (1998). Maternal and Child Health Research Consortium, 188 Baker Street, London.

4. Department of Health; Welsh Office; Scottish Office Home and Health Department; Department of Health and Social Services, Northern Ireland (1996). Report on Confidential Enquiries into Maternal Deaths in the United Kingdom 1991-1993. London, HMSO.

5. Department of Health. Why Mothers Die. Report on Confidential Enquiries into Maternal Deaths in the United Kingdom 1994-1996. (1998). TSO, London.

6. NHS Management Executive. Hours of work of doctors in training: working arrangements of doctors and dentists in training. In: Junior Doctors - the New Deal (1991). NHS Management Executive.

7. Honour P. Review of the Maternity Services 1996/97 - District Audit. Southampton.

8. Changing Childbirth: Report of the Expert Maternity Group (1993). HMSO, London.

9. UKCC. Statistical analysis of the UKCC's professional register 1 April 1997 to 31 March 1998 (1998). UKCC, London pp 9-14.

10. UKCC. Guidelines for records and record keeping (1998). UKCC, London.

11. RCM Position Paper 2 Safety in Maternity Units (1994). RCM, London.

12. Garcia J, Redshaw M, Fitzsimons B, Keene J. First Class Delivery. A national survey of women's views of maternity care (1998). Audit Commission Publications, Abingdon, Oxon.

13. Recommended minimum standards for obstetric anaesthesia services (1998). Obstetric Anaesthetists Association, Secretary OAA, Nottingham City Hospital, Nottingham NG5 1PB.

14. Ball, J. Birthrate (1992).

15. Department of Health. A First Class Service: Quality in the new NHS (1998). Department of Health, London.

16. Assistance for the Anaesthetist (1988). Association of Anaesthetists of Great Britain and Ireland, London.

17. Neonatal Resuscitation. The Report of a BPA Working Party (1993). British Paediatric Association, London.

18. Training needs of professionals responsible for resuscitation of babies at birth (1998). RCOG/RCPCH. RCOG. London.

19. UKCC. Midwives Rules and Code of Practice (1998). UKCC, London.

20. Flint C. Know your Midwife. Continuity of care provided by a team of midwives. (1993). In Midwives, Research and Childbirth Vol II (eds. Robinson S and Thomson A). Chapman Hall. pp 72-103.

21. Oakley A. Is social support good for the health of mothers and babies? (1988). Journal of Reproductive and Infant Psychology 6: 3-21.

22. UKCC. Rule 40 - Responsibility and sphere of Practice. In: Midwives Rules and Code of Practice. (1998) UKCC, London.

23. Advanced Life Support in Obstetrics (ALSO)(1996). ALSO UK, Newcastle upon Tyne. (0191 256 3281).

24. Wilkinson C, McIlwaine G, Boulton-Jones C, Cole S (1998). Is a rising Caesarean section rate inevitable? *Br J Obstet Gynaecol* **105**, 45-52.

25. Stewart J H, Andrews J, Cartlidge P H T (1998). Numbers of deaths related to intrapartum asphyxia and timing of birth in all Wales perinatal survey 1993-5. *B Med J* **316**, 657-660.

26. ENB Supervision of Midwives (1996). London.

27. Monitoring Good Medical Practice (1998). General Medical Council, London.

28. Mitchell T (1995). CTG - A Guidance for Interpretation - The Crimson File. A selection of cases compiled during a confidential inquiry. West Midlands Perinatal Audit, Solihull.

29. Disability Discrimination Act (1995).

30. Cordingley J J, Rubin A P (1997). A survey of facilities for high risk women in consultant obstetric units. *International Journal of Obstetric Anesthesia* **6**; 156-160.

31. Audit Commission. First Class Delivery. Improving Maternity Services in England and Wales (1997). Audit Commission Publications, Abingdon, Oxon.

32. Resuscitation of Babies at Birth (1997). Report of Joint Committee RCOG/RCPCH. BMJ Publishing, London.

33. RCM Evidence to the Review Body for Nursing Staff, Midwives, Health Visitors and Professions allied to Medicine for 1999 (1998). RCM, London.

Risk Management Standard Number 11

Reproduced from Clinical Negligence Scheme for Trusts Manual of Risk
Management Standards   (August 1997 Version 1)

Standard:

**There is a clear documented system for management and
communication throughout the key stages of maternity**

Rationale:

*The majority of costly claims arise in the field of Obstetrics. Clinical
risk management therefore requires specific attention in this area.*

**NB. In view of the changing nature of maternity care, we envisage
changes and extensions to these Standards over the next year or so -
particularly at level three.**

Areas for assessment:

Standard 11   Level

1.1   The arrangements are clear concerning which professional   [1]
        is responsible for the care at all times

        (Guidelines for ante-natal booking, case-notes)

1.2   The professional responsible for intrapartum care is clearly   [1]
        identified

        (Labour Ward guidelines)

1.3   There are detailed multi-disciplinary policies for management   [1]
        of all key conditions / situations on the labour ward.

        *(e.g.. Diabetes, Severe Hypertension, shoulder Dystocia, Water Birth,
        Ruptured Uterus. For the complete list see the "Topic Summary" at the
        end of this manual.)*

        (Maternity/Labour Ward guidelines)

1.4   There is an agreed mechanism for direct referral to a consultant   [1]
       from a midwife

1.5   There is a personal handover of care when medical or   [1]
       midwifery shifts change

       (Copy of protocol; medical staff handbook)

2.1   There is a named consultant with designated responsibility   [2]
       for maternity/labour ward matters

2.2   There is clear guidance on the transfer of care during the   [2]
       intrapartum period

3.1   A doctor of at least 12 months' obstetrics experience should be   [3]
       resident on the labour ward at all times, or available within
       5 minutes.

       A doctor of at least three years' experience in obstetrics should be
       available within 30 minutes.

       (Relevant timetable/job plan)

3.2   The delivery interval in CS for fetal distress is subject to an
       annually audited standard.

       (Standard, and audit documents)

3.3   There is a personal handover to obstetric locums, either by   [3]
       post-holder, or senior member of the team, and vice-versa.

       (Policy document and procedure)

Birthrate

In 1991 both the Royal College of Obstetricians and Gynaecologists and the Royal College of Midwives recommended Birthrate to the House of Commons Select Committee on Maternity Care as a rational basis for assessing staffing needs in delivery units.

Birthrate has three main components:

1. Score system

    Five different categories of maternal and neonatal outcome are created by the score system. The lower the score, the more normal are the processes of labour and delivery. Increasing degrees of intervention or support are reflected in the higher categories. Although Category V will include many cases of emergency caesarean section, it has also been found to include those women who achieve a normal delivery and healthy baby following high levels of support during labour (eg diabetic women) and those who experience unexpected complications with the baby, or for the mother post-delivery.

2. Midwife hours

    Midwife hours per woman category are based upon the standards recommended in the Short Report (1980) and the Maternity Care in Action Report on Intrapartum Care (1985), namely that women should be attended by a midwife throughout labour.

3. Staffing formula

    A staffing formula then converts the data into the number of midwives required to meet the measured workload and standards of care.

References

Social Services Committee: Fourth Report: Session 1980-81. Medical Education. (1980). (The Short Report) HMSO, London.

Maternity Care in Action Part II. Care during Childbirth (Intrapartum Care) (1984).
HMSO, London.

Ball, J.A., Dependency levels in delivery suites: Proceedings of the Research and the Midwife Conference 1988.

Ball, J.A., (1989). Birthrate: A method of outcome review and manpower planning in the delivery suite. Nuffield Institute for Health Services Studies. University of Leeds.

Neonatal Resuscitation Equipment

Extracted from Resuscitation of Babies at Birth (1997), a Report of the Royal College of Paediatrics and Child Health and the Royal College of Obstetricians and Gynaecologists published by BMJ Publishing Group

Equipment for resuscitation at home

Access to a mobile phone or telephone within the home
A room heater and good light
An appropriate padded surface at table height
Towels and gloves
Self-inflating resuscitation bag, valve and face masks of different sizes
Suction device and catheters
Resuscitation flow chart
Stop watch
Stethoscope
Oxygen cylinder with regulated flow rate of up to 10 L/min and an adjustable pressure-relief valve within the system
Syringes, needles and disposal box
Checklist

Equipment for resuscitation in hospital

This is a suggested list of what should be available in each delivery room and in the accident and emergency department:

A resuscitation surface
An overhead radiant heat source
Towels and gloves
Stop clock
Stethoscope
Suction device and catheters
Oxygen/air supply with variable regulated flow rate and adjustable pressure-relief valve
Y-piece or 500-ml self-inflating resuscitation bag, valve and face masks
Two laryngoscopes with straight, appropriate size blades, spare bulbs and batteries
Tracheal tubes (2.5, 3.0 and 4.0 mm), introducers and connectors
Magill forceps if using nasal route for intubation
Syringes
Scissors
Adhesive tape
Umbilical vessel catheterisation pack
Nasogastric tube sizes 5 and 8
Oropharyngeal airways, sizes 00 and 0
Intravenous cannulae
Pleural cannula set
Checklist
Resuscitation Charts 1 and 2

Auditable Standards   Source

1 A standing labour ward committee exists   RCOG MSL

2 Guidelines/protocols for intrapartum care are available   RCOG OSMS

3 The date such guidelines were established should be   RCOG OSMS
   recorded and they should be reviewed at least every 3
   years

4 A minimum consultant supervision for the labour ward   CNST
   should be 40 hours, unless the unit delivers less than 1000
   babies/year

5 Junior staffing levels will depend on training opportunities RCOG Higher
                                                                 Training Cttee

6 Midwifery staffing should provide 1.15/1 midwives/   Audit
   woman in normal labour   Commission

7 Alternatively 75% of women should have the same   RCOG OSMS
   midwife throughout their labour

8 There should be documented evidence of a consultant   RCOG MSL
   ward round at least twice during the day and once during
   the evening

9 There should be documented evidence that the consultant   RCOG MSL
   is being contacted prior to emergency caesarean section or
   when a patient's condition gives rise for concern

10 Ten per cent of complicated deliveries should be attended   RCOG OSMS
   by a consultant

11 Medical staffing levels on labour wards should be audited   RCOG OSMS

   a)   A doctor of at least 12 months' experience should be
        resident on labour ward, or available within 5 minutes.

   b)   A doctor of at least 3 years' obstetric experience
        should be available within 30 minutes.

12 Anaesthetic cover should be audited   RCOG OSMS

   a)   An anaesthetist with at least one year's experience
        should be available within 10 minutes.

   b)   The anaesthetic response time should be such that a
        caesarean section could be started within 30 minutes
        of the decision to proceed.

   c)   All women requiring conduction or general anaesthesia
        should be visited by an anaesthetist before an elective
        procedure.

d) Over 80% of women having a caesarean section, on the assumption that those offered will accept, should be offered a regional block.

e) A named consultant should be responsible for ensuring standards for obstetric analgesia and resuscitation.

f) Staff should be "drilled" to cope with acute obstetric emergencies.

13 The following outcomes should be recorded

Emergency caesarean sections, incidence and indications	OQIRD
Percentage of labours lasting >18 hours	OQIRD
Apgar scores , < 7 at 5 minutes	OQIRD
Need for neonatal resuscitation	OQIRD
Admissions to special care for babies weighing greater than 2.5 kg	OQIRD
Intrapartum stillbirths	OQIRD
Incidence of primary postpartum haemorrhage	OQIRD
Total deliveries	RCOG OSMS
Inductions, indications and outcomes	RCOG OSMS
Augmentation of labour	RCOG OSMS
Instrumental delivery rates - ventouse, forceps	RCOG OSMS
Elective caesarean section rates and indications	RCOG OSMS
Episiotomy rates	RCOG OSMS
Epidural rates	RCOG OSMS
Breast feeding rates	RCOG OSMS
% of complicated deliveries attended by consultant	RCOG MSL

14 All clinical staff involved with care in labour should attend management of labour/CTG refresher courses every six months (arranged locally). A personal log book of attendances should be kept.   RCOG MSL

15 A weekly review of labour ward cases and CTGs should be established attended by both medical and midwifery staff.   RCOG MSL

16 Labour ward facilities should be at an appropriate standard; facilities for bereaved parents should be available.   RCOG OSMS

Sources

CNST   Clinical Negligence Scheme for Trusts

OQIRD   Obstetric Quality Indicators from Routine Data. King's Fund Comparative Initiative (1997). CASPE.

RCOG MSL   Minimum Standards of Care in Labour 1994

RCOG OSMS   Organisational Standards for Maternity Services (1995)